PEPTIDES FOR HEALTH AND WELLNESS

A COMPREHENSIVE GUIDE TO USING PEPTIDE THERAPIES FOR CHRONIC PAIN, INFLAMMATION AND AGING

Katherine Peters

Table of Contents

Introduction

The world of health and wellness is constantly evolving, driven by new scientific discoveries and technological advancements. One of the most exciting and promising areas of development in recent years is the field of peptide therapies. As researchers uncover the vast potential of peptides to address various health issues, there has been a surge of interest and enthusiasm from both the scientific community and the general public. "Peptides for Health and Wellness: A Comprehensive Guide to Using Peptide Therapies for Chronic Pain, Inflammation, and Aging" aims to demystify this complex yet fascinating topic, offering readers an in-depth understanding of how peptides can revolutionize their approach to health and wellness.

The Promise of Peptide Therapies

Peptides have emerged as a powerful tool in the quest for better health. These short chains of amino acids are the building blocks of proteins and play crucial roles in a multitude of biological processes. The unique properties of peptides make them particularly promising for therapeutic applications. Unlike larger proteins, peptides are small enough to easily penetrate cell membranes and can be engineered to interact with specific targets within the body, offering a high degree of precision in treatment.

In recent years, the popularity of peptide therapies has skyrocketed. This surge can be attributed to several factors. First, there is a growing body of scientific evidence supporting the efficacy of peptides in treating a range of conditions, from chronic pain and inflammation to the signs of aging. Additionally, advances in biotechnology have made it easier and more cost-effective to produce synthetic peptides, making these therapies more accessible to the public.

One of the most compelling aspects of peptide therapies is their potential to address the root causes of health issues rather than merely alleviating symptoms. For instance, certain peptides can modulate immune responses, reduce inflammation at its source, and promote tissue repair and regeneration. This holistic approach not only improves overall health but also enhances the body's natural ability to heal itself.

A Brief History of Peptide Research

The journey of peptide research is marked by several key milestones that have paved the way for the current advancements in peptide therapies. The discovery of peptides dates back to the early 20th century when scientists first identified these molecules as essential components of proteins. However, it wasn't until the mid-20th century that the therapeutic potential of peptides began to be explored in earnest.

One of the pivotal moments in peptide research came in 1953 when Frederick Sanger determined the amino acid sequence of insulin, a peptide hormone. This groundbreaking work not only earned Sanger a Nobel Prize but also demonstrated the immense potential of peptides in regulating biological processes. Over the following decades, researchers continued to explore the roles of various peptides in the body, leading to the identification of numerous peptide hormones, neurotransmitters, and signaling molecules.

The development of synthetic peptides in the latter half of the 20th century marked another significant milestone. Advances in peptide synthesis techniques allowed scientists to create peptides with specific sequences and properties, opening up new possibilities for therapeutic applications. Notable researchers, such as Bruce Merrifield, who developed solid-phase peptide synthesis, revolutionized the field and earned a Nobel Prize for his contributions.

In recent years, the focus of peptide research has shifted towards understanding the mechanisms of action of therapeutic peptides and developing novel delivery systems to enhance their efficacy and safety. Clinical trials and real-world applications have provided valuable insights into the benefits and challenges of peptide therapies, further solidifying their place in modern medicine.

Overview of the Book

"Peptides for Health and Wellness: A Comprehensive Guide to Using Peptide Therapies for Chronic Pain, Inflammation, and Aging" is designed to be a comprehensive and accessible resource for anyone interested in exploring the potential of peptide therapies.

Whether you are a healthcare professional looking to expand your knowledge, a patient seeking alternative treatment options, or simply a curious reader, this book will provide you with valuable insights and practical guidance.

The book is structured to take you on a journey from the basic concepts of peptides to their advanced therapeutic applications. It begins with an introduction to the world of peptides, explaining what they are, how they work in the body, and their significance in various biological processes. This foundational knowledge sets the stage for the more detailed discussions that follow.

By bridging the gap between cutting-edge science and practical application, "Peptides for Health and Wellness" aims to empower readers with the knowledge and tools to harness the potential of peptide therapies for a healthier, more vibrant life.

Chapter 1

Understanding Peptides

Peptides have emerged as significant players in the health and wellness industry, attracting attention for their vast therapeutic potential. This chapter explores the fundamental nature of peptides, elucidating their structure, biological roles, and the vital functions they serve in maintaining health and homeostasis.

What Are Peptides?

Peptides are short chains of amino acids linked by peptide bonds. Each peptide bond forms when the carboxyl group of one amino acid reacts with the amino group of another, releasing a molecule of water in the process. The resulting structure is a linear sequence of amino acids that can range from as few as two to several dozen in length.

At their core, peptides are composed of the same building blocks as proteins: amino acids. However, the distinction between peptides and proteins lies primarily in their size and complexity. Peptides are generally shorter and less complex than proteins, typically containing fewer than 50 amino acids. Proteins, on the other hand, can be composed of hundreds or even thousands of amino acids, often folding into intricate three-dimensional structures essential for their function.

The basic structure of a peptide can be represented as follows:

1. **N-Terminus**: The end of the peptide chain with a free amino group (-NH2).

2. **C-Terminus**: The end of the peptide chain with a free carboxyl group (-COOH).

3. **Amino Acid Sequence**: The linear sequence of amino acids, each linked by peptide bonds.

This simple yet versatile structure allows peptides to perform a wide array of functions within the body, acting as signaling molecules, hormones, enzymes, and more.

Differentiating Peptides from Proteins and Other Biological Molecules

While peptides and proteins share a common composition of amino acids, they differ significantly in terms of size, structure, and function. Proteins are typically much larger than peptides and fold into specific three-dimensional shapes that are crucial for their function. This folding is driven by various interactions between the amino acids in the protein chain, including hydrogen bonds, hydrophobic interactions, and disulfide bridges.

Proteins are involved in virtually every biological process within the body. They act as enzymes catalyzing biochemical reactions, structural components providing support and shape to cells, transporters carrying molecules across cell membranes, and antibodies defending against pathogens.

In contrast, peptides are shorter and often act as signaling molecules or hormones. Their smaller size allows them to diffuse more readily through tissues and interact with specific receptors on the surface of cells, triggering various biological responses. This ability to act as messengers and regulators makes peptides particularly valuable in therapeutic applications.

Other biological molecules, such as nucleic acids (DNA and RNA), lipids, and carbohydrates, differ from peptides and proteins in both structure and function. Nucleic acids store and transmit genetic information, lipids form the structural basis of cell membranes and store energy, and carbohydrates provide energy and serve as structural components. Each of these classes of molecules plays a unique and essential role in maintaining the life and function of cells and organisms.

How Peptides Work in the Body

Peptides serve as crucial regulators of numerous physiological processes within the body. They act as messengers, transmitting signals between cells, tissues, and organs to coordinate and regulate biological activities. Some of the key roles peptides play include:

1. **Cell Signaling**: Peptides function as signaling molecules that bind to specific receptors on the surface of target cells, initiating a cascade of cellular responses. This signaling can influence various processes, including cell growth, differentiation, and metabolism.

2. **Hormone Regulation**: Many hormones are peptides or proteins that regulate essential bodily functions. For example, insulin, a peptide hormone produced by the pancreas, regulates blood sugar levels by facilitating the uptake of glucose into cells.

3. **Immune Responses**: Peptides are integral to the functioning of the immune system. They can act as antimicrobial agents, targeting and neutralizing pathogens, or as immunomodulators, influencing the activity of immune cells.

4. **Neurotransmission**: Certain peptides function as neurotransmitters or neuromodulators in the nervous system. They transmit signals between neurons, affecting mood, behavior, and cognitive functions.

Examples of Naturally Occurring Peptides and Their Functions

Several naturally occurring peptides play vital roles in maintaining health and regulating physiological processes. Here are a few notable examples:

1. **Insulin**: As mentioned earlier, insulin is a peptide hormone that regulates blood glucose levels. It facilitates the uptake of glucose by cells, thereby lowering blood sugar levels and providing energy for cellular activities.

2. **Oxytocin**: Often referred to as the "love hormone," oxytocin is a peptide that plays a crucial role in social bonding, reproduction, and childbirth. It promotes feelings of trust, empathy, and social connection.

3. **Glucagon**: This peptide hormone works in opposition to insulin. It stimulates the liver to convert stored glycogen into glucose, releasing it into the bloodstream to raise blood sugar levels when they are too low.

4. **Vasopressin**: Also known as antidiuretic hormone (ADH), vasopressin regulates water balance in the body by increasing the reabsorption of water in the kidneys, thereby reducing urine output and conserving water.

5. **Substance P**: This neuropeptide is involved in transmitting pain signals from peripheral nerves to the central nervous system. It plays a role in the perception of pain and the inflammatory response.

6. **Endorphins**: These peptides act as natural painkillers and mood enhancers. They are released in response to stress, pain, or exercise and help alleviate pain and induce feelings of euphoria.

These examples illustrate the diverse and essential functions that peptides perform within the body, highlighting their importance in maintaining health and well-being.

The Role of Peptides in Biological Processes

Peptides play a pivotal role in various biological processes, acting as key regulators and facilitators of cellular communication and function. Their ability to influence cell signaling, hormone regulation, and immune responses underscores their significance in maintaining health and homeostasis.

1. **Cell Signaling**: Peptides are critical components of cell signaling pathways. When a peptide binds to a specific receptor on the surface of a target cell, it triggers a series of intracellular events that lead to a specific response. This process, known as signal transduction, can result in changes

in gene expression, enzyme activity, or cellular behavior. For example, the peptide hormone insulin binds to its receptor on the surface of muscle and fat cells, triggering a cascade of events that lead to the uptake of glucose and the regulation of blood sugar levels.

2. **Hormone Regulation**: Hormones are chemical messengers that regulate various physiological processes. Many hormones are peptides or proteins, and they exert their effects by binding to specific receptors on target cells. For instance, thyroid-stimulating hormone (TSH) is a peptide hormone that stimulates the thyroid gland to produce thyroid hormones, which regulate metabolism, growth, and development. The precise regulation of hormone levels and their interactions with receptors are essential for maintaining homeostasis.

3. **Immune Responses**: Peptides play a crucial role in the immune system, acting as signaling molecules that coordinate the activity of immune cells. For example, cytokines are a group of peptides that regulate the immune

response by promoting or inhibiting the activity of various immune cells. Antimicrobial peptides, such as defensins, are produced by the body as part of the innate immune response and can directly kill bacteria, viruses, and fungi. Peptides also function as antigens, stimulating the production of antibodies by the immune system to protect against infections.

The Importance of Peptides in Maintaining Homeostasis and Health

Homeostasis refers to the body's ability to maintain a stable internal environment despite external fluctuations. Peptides are essential in maintaining homeostasis by regulating a wide range of physiological processes. Their roles in cell signaling, hormone regulation, and immune responses illustrate their critical contributions to overall health.

1. **Regulation of Metabolism**: Peptides such as insulin and glucagon play a central role in regulating metabolism and maintaining blood sugar levels. Insulin promotes the uptake

and storage of glucose, while glucagon stimulates the release of glucose from the liver. Together, these peptides ensure that energy is available when needed and that blood sugar levels remain within a narrow range.

2. **Fluid and Electrolyte Balance**: Peptide hormones like vasopressin and atrial natriuretic peptide (ANP) regulate fluid and electrolyte balance in the body. Vasopressin increases water reabsorption in the kidneys, reducing urine output and conserving water. ANP, on the other hand, promotes the excretion of sodium and water, helping to reduce blood pressure and maintain fluid balance.

3. **Stress Response**: Peptides are involved in the body's response to stress. For example, corticotropin-releasing hormone (CRH) is a peptide that stimulates the release of adrenocorticotropic hormone (ACTH) from the pituitary gland, which in turn triggers the production of cortisol by the adrenal glands. Cortisol helps the body cope with stress by mobilizing energy reserves and modulating immune responses.

4. **Growth and Development**: Peptides such as growth hormone (GH) and insulin-like growth factors (IGFs) are crucial for growth and development. GH stimulates the growth of bones and tissues, while IGFs mediate many of the growth-promoting effects of GH. These peptides are essential for normal growth during childhood and for maintaining tissue health and repair in adults.

5. **Reproductive Health**: Peptide hormones like gonadotropin-releasing hormone (GnRH) and oxytocin play key roles in reproductive health. GnRH regulates the release of other hormones involved in reproductive processes, such as luteinizing hormone (LH) and follicle-stimulating hormone (FSH). These hormones are critical for the regulation of the menstrual cycle, ovulation, and sperm production. Oxytocin, as mentioned earlier, is essential for childbirth and lactation, as well as fostering social bonding and emotional connections.

6. **Pain Management and Mood Regulation**: Endorphins, often referred to as the body's natural painkillers, are peptides that interact with opioid receptors in the brain to reduce the perception of pain. They are released in response to stress, pain, and physical exercise, contributing to the sensation of well-being and euphoria. Similarly, peptides like substance P are involved in transmitting pain signals and regulating inflammatory responses, highlighting their dual role in both pain perception and immune function.

Peptides, through their diverse and critical roles, underscore their significance in maintaining homeostasis and overall health. By modulating various physiological processes, peptides ensure that the body can adapt to changes and maintain equilibrium, thus promoting health and preventing disease.

Chapter 2

The Science Behind Peptide Therapies

Peptide therapies have emerged as a promising frontier in modern medicine, offering targeted treatments with the potential for fewer side effects compared to conventional drugs. This chapter delves into the science behind peptide therapies, exploring how peptides interact with biological systems, the key research that supports their efficacy, and the innovations in peptide delivery that enhance their therapeutic potential.

The Mechanisms of Peptide Action

Peptides Interact with Receptors and Cells in the Body

Peptides exert their effects primarily through their interactions with specific receptors on the surfaces of cells. These receptors are proteins that recognize and bind to peptides with high specificity, much like a lock and key mechanism. When a peptide binds to its receptor, it triggers a series of intracellular events that result in a physiological response. This process is known as signal transduction.

The interaction between a peptide and its receptor can initiate various cellular processes, depending on the type of receptor and the cellular context. Some common pathways influenced by peptide-receptor interactions include:

1. **G-Protein Coupled Receptors (GPCRs):** Many peptides bind to GPCRs, which are a large family of receptors involved in numerous physiological processes. When a peptide binds to a GPCR, it activates an associated G-protein, which then triggers downstream signaling pathways. These pathways can lead to changes in gene expression, enzyme activity, or cellular behavior.

2. **Tyrosine Kinase Receptors**: Some peptides, like insulin, bind to receptors that possess intrinsic tyrosine

kinase activity. Upon peptide binding, these receptors undergo autophosphorylation, activating kinase activity that initiates a cascade of phosphorylation events inside the cell. This cascade can influence cell growth, differentiation, metabolism, and survival.

3. **Ion Channel Receptors**: Certain peptides interact with ion channel receptors, which control the flow of ions across cell membranes. Binding of the peptide can cause the ion channel to open or close, altering the cell's electrical activity and affecting processes like neurotransmission, muscle contraction, and hormone secretion.

Biochemical Pathways Influenced by Peptide Therapies.

Peptides can modulate a wide range of biochemical pathways, each contributing to their therapeutic effects. Some key pathways influenced by peptide therapies include:

1. **Insulin Signaling Pathway**: Insulin, a peptide hormone, binds to its receptor on target cells, activating the insulin receptor tyrosine kinase. This activation triggers a cascade involving insulin receptor substrates (IRS) and phosphatidylinositol 3-kinase (PI3K), leading to the activation of protein kinase B (Akt). Akt promotes glucose uptake by translocating glucose transporter 4 (GLUT4) to the cell membrane, thereby lowering blood glucose levels.

2. **cAMP Pathway**: Many peptides, such as glucagon and parathyroid hormone, activate GPCRs that stimulate adenylate cyclase, an enzyme that converts ATP to cyclic AMP (cAMP). cAMP acts as a second messenger, activating protein kinase A (PKA), which phosphorylates various target proteins to regulate processes like glycogen breakdown, lipolysis, and gene transcription.

3. **MAPK/ERK Pathway**: Peptides like growth factors activate the mitogen-activated protein kinase (MAPK) pathway. This pathway involves a series of kinases, including MAPK/ERK kinase (MEK) and extracellular

signal-regulated kinase (ERK), which ultimately lead to changes in gene expression that promote cell proliferation, differentiation, and survival.

4. **JAK/STAT Pathway**: Cytokines, a class of signaling peptides, often activate the Janus kinase (JAK)/signal transducer and activator of transcription (STAT) pathway. Binding of a cytokine to its receptor activates JAK, which phosphorylates and activates STAT proteins. STATs then translocate to the nucleus to regulate gene expression, influencing immune responses and inflammation.

By modulating these and other biochemical pathways, peptide therapies can effectively target specific physiological processes, offering precise treatments for various health conditions.

The therapeutic potential of peptides has been supported by numerous landmark studies. Here are a few significant examples:

1. **Insulin for Diabetes Management**: The discovery and development of insulin therapy for diabetes is one of the most well-known and impactful examples of peptide therapy. In the early 1920s, Frederick Banting and Charles Best demonstrated that extracts from the pancreas could lower blood sugar levels in diabetic dogs. This discovery led to the first successful use of insulin in humans, revolutionizing the treatment of diabetes and saving millions of lives.

2. **GLP-1 Analogs for Diabetes**: Glucagon-like peptide-1 (GLP-1) is a peptide hormone that enhances insulin

secretion and inhibits glucagon release. Research led to the development of GLP-1 analogs, such as exenatide and liraglutide, which have been shown to improve glycemic control in patients with type 2 diabetes. These therapies mimic the action of GLP-1, providing significant benefits in glucose regulation and weight management.

3. **BPC-157 for Tissue Repair**: Body Protection Compound-157 (BPC-157) is a synthetic peptide derived from a protective protein found in the stomach. Studies have shown that BPC-157 can promote healing and tissue repair in various models of injury, including tendon, muscle, and nerve damage. Research indicates that BPC-157 may enhance angiogenesis (formation of new blood vessels) and modulate inflammation, making it a promising candidate for regenerative medicine.

Scientific Evidence Supporting the Use of Peptides for Health Conditions.

The scientific evidence supporting peptide therapies spans various health conditions, demonstrating their versatility and potential. Here are some key areas where peptides have shown significant promise:

1. **Chronic Pain and Inflammation**: Peptides like substance P and enkephalins are involved in pain signaling and modulation. Research has shown that certain peptide-based treatments can alleviate chronic pain and reduce inflammation. For example, enkephalin analogs have been investigated for their potential to manage pain without the side effects associated with traditional opioids.

2. **Anti-Aging and Skin Health**: Peptides like collagen peptides and matrixyl have gained popularity for their anti-aging properties. Collagen peptides can improve skin elasticity and hydration by stimulating collagen production, while matrixyl peptides promote the synthesis of

extracellular matrix components. Clinical studies have demonstrated that these peptides can reduce wrinkles and improve overall skin appearance.

3. **Cancer Therapy**: Peptide-based cancer therapies are an area of active research. Certain peptides can target cancer cells with high specificity, delivering cytotoxic agents directly to the tumor. For instance, peptide-drug conjugates (PDCs) combine peptides with chemotherapeutic agents, allowing for targeted delivery and reducing off-target effects. Peptides like somatostatin analogs are also used to treat neuroendocrine tumors by inhibiting hormone secretion and tumor growth.

4. **Cardiovascular Health**: Peptides such as natriuretic peptides (e.g., BNP and ANP) play a role in cardiovascular regulation by promoting vasodilation and reducing blood pressure. Clinical studies have explored the use of natriuretic peptides in managing heart failure, demonstrating their potential to improve cardiac function and reduce symptoms.

These examples underscore the diverse applications of peptide therapies and the robust scientific evidence supporting their efficacy.

Innovations in Peptide Delivery Systems

One of the challenges in peptide therapy is ensuring that peptides are delivered effectively and safely to their target sites. Peptides are susceptible to degradation by enzymes and may have limited bioavailability when administered orally. To address these challenges, several innovative delivery systems have been developed:

1. **Injectable Peptides**: Injectable delivery remains one of the most common and effective methods for administering peptides. Subcutaneous, intramuscular, and intravenous injections can bypass the digestive system, ensuring that peptides reach the bloodstream intact. Advances in

formulation and stabilization have improved the efficacy and patient compliance of injectable peptides.

2. **Transdermal Systems**: Transdermal delivery systems, such as patches and gels, offer a non-invasive alternative for peptide administration. These systems enable the controlled release of peptides through the skin, providing a steady and prolonged therapeutic effect. Techniques like microneedles and iontophoresis (using electric current) enhance the penetration of peptides through the skin barrier.

3. **Oral Peptides**: Developing oral peptide therapies has been a significant focus of research. Efforts to improve the stability and absorption of oral peptides include the use of enzyme inhibitors, permeation enhancers, and nanoparticle encapsulation. For example, oral formulations of GLP-1 analogs have been developed, showing promise in managing diabetes with the convenience of oral administration.

4. **Intranasal Delivery**: Intranasal delivery offers a rapid and direct route for peptides to enter the systemic circulation and the central nervous system. This method bypasses the blood-brain barrier, making it suitable for delivering peptides that target neurological conditions. Intranasal oxytocin, for instance, has been explored for its potential in treating social and anxiety disorders.

5. **Peptide Conjugates**: Peptide conjugation involves linking peptides to other molecules, such as antibodies or polymers, to enhance their stability, targeting, and efficacy. Antibody-peptide conjugates (APCs) combine the specificity of antibodies with the therapeutic effects of peptides, allowing for targeted delivery to cancer cells or other disease sites. Polymer conjugation can improve the solubility and half-life of peptides, extending their therapeutic action.

Chapter 3

Peptides for Chronic Pain Relief

Chronic pain affects millions of people worldwide, significantly diminishing their quality of life. Despite advancements in conventional treatments, many patients continue to suffer from persistent pain that is difficult to manage. Peptide therapies offer a novel and promising approach to chronic pain relief, targeting pain mechanisms with precision and potentially providing more effective and longer-lasting relief. In this chapter, we explore the common types of chronic pain, the limitations of current treatments, and how peptides can offer new hope for those suffering from chronic pain.

Common Types of Chronic Pain

Chronic pain is defined as pain that persists for longer than three months, often beyond the expected period of healing.

It can arise from various underlying conditions and can be broadly categorized into several types:

1. **Neuropathic Pain**: This type of pain results from damage or dysfunction in the nervous system. Common causes include diabetes (diabetic neuropathy), shingles (postherpetic neuralgia), and nerve injuries. Neuropathic pain is often described as burning, stabbing, or shooting and can be accompanied by numbness and tingling. Traditional treatments, such as anticonvulsants and antidepressants, often provide limited relief and can have significant side effects.

2. **Arthritis**: Arthritis is a leading cause of chronic pain, affecting joints and surrounding tissues. Osteoarthritis, the most common form, is caused by the degeneration of cartilage, leading to pain, stiffness, and reduced mobility. Rheumatoid arthritis, an autoimmune disorder, results in inflammation of the joints, causing severe pain and deformity. Conventional treatments, including NSAIDs and disease-modifying antirheumatic drugs (DMARDs), may

not fully alleviate pain and can have adverse effects with long-term use.

3. **Fibromyalgia**: Characterized by widespread musculoskeletal pain, fibromyalgia is often accompanied by fatigue, sleep disturbances, and cognitive difficulties. The exact cause is unknown, but it is believed to involve abnormal pain processing in the central nervous system. Treatment typically involves a combination of medications, such as pain relievers and antidepressants, and lifestyle modifications, which may not provide complete relief.

4. **Chronic Back Pain**: One of the most common reasons for medical visits, chronic back pain can result from various causes, including degenerative disc disease, spinal stenosis, and muscle or ligament strain. Pain can range from a dull ache to a sharp, debilitating sensation. Standard treatments include physical therapy, pain medications, and in severe cases, surgery, but many patients continue to experience persistent pain.

5. **Migraine**: Migraines are severe headaches often accompanied by nausea, vomiting, and sensitivity to light and sound. They can last for hours to days and significantly

impact daily functioning. While preventive and acute treatments are available, many patients find them inadequate in managing the frequency and intensity of migraines.

Chronic pain can have profound effects on an individual's physical, emotional, and social well-being. It can limit mobility, interfere with daily activities, and reduce overall productivity. The constant struggle with pain can lead to mental health issues such as depression and anxiety, creating a vicious cycle that exacerbates the perception of pain.

The limitations of conventional treatments for chronic pain are significant. Many pain medications, such as opioids, can be highly effective in the short term but carry a risk of addiction and tolerance, leading to decreased effectiveness over time. Nonsteroidal anti-inflammatory drugs (NSAIDs) and other analgesics can cause gastrointestinal, cardiovascular, and renal side effects with long-term use. Furthermore, many standard treatments do not address the underlying causes of pain or modulate the complex pathways involved in chronic pain syndromes.

Given these challenges, there is a pressing need for new, targeted therapies that can provide sustained pain relief with minimal side effects. Peptides, with their ability to specifically target pain mechanisms, offer a promising solution.

Peptides can alleviate pain through various mechanisms, targeting specific pathways involved in pain signaling and modulation. Some of the key mechanisms include:

1. **Modulation of Neurotransmitter Release**: Peptides can influence the release of neurotransmitters involved in pain transmission. For example, enkephalins are endogenous peptides that bind to opioid receptors, inhibiting the release

of substance P, a neurotransmitter that facilitates pain signaling. By reducing substance P levels, enkephalins can decrease pain perception.

2. **Blocking Pain Receptors**: Certain peptides can directly block pain receptors, preventing the transmission of pain signals. For instance, conotoxins, derived from the venom of marine cone snails, can inhibit voltage-gated calcium channels on nerve cells. This blockade prevents the release of pain-inducing neurotransmitters, effectively reducing pain.

3. **Anti-Inflammatory Effects**: Many peptides exhibit anti-inflammatory properties, which can help alleviate pain associated with inflammation. For example, BPC-157, a synthetic peptide, has been shown to reduce inflammation by modulating the production of pro-inflammatory cytokines. By decreasing inflammation, these peptides can alleviate pain and promote healing.

4. **Nerve Regeneration and Repair**: Peptides can also promote the repair and regeneration of damaged nerves, addressing the root cause of neuropathic pain. Thymosin beta-4, for example, has been found to enhance nerve regeneration by promoting the migration and differentiation of nerve cells. This regenerative effect can help restore normal function and reduce pain.

5. **Central Sensitization Modulation**: Chronic pain often involves central sensitization, a state where the central nervous system becomes hypersensitive to pain stimuli. Peptides can modulate this process by targeting receptors and signaling pathways involved in central sensitization. For instance, peptides that activate the inhibitory gamma-aminobutyric acid (GABA) receptors can dampen the heightened pain response.

Several peptides have shown promise in pain management through their unique modes of action. Some notable examples include:

1. **Enkephalins**: These endogenous opioid peptides bind to opioid receptors in the central and peripheral nervous systems, inhibiting pain signaling. Enkephalins reduce the release of substance P and other pain-related neurotransmitters, providing analgesic effects similar to those of morphine but without the risk of addiction and tolerance.

2. **Conotoxins**: Derived from the venom of cone snails, conotoxins are potent inhibitors of voltage-gated calcium channels. By blocking these channels, conotoxins prevent the release of neurotransmitters involved in pain transmission. Ziconotide, a synthetic conotoxin, has been approved for the treatment of severe chronic pain, particularly in patients who do not respond to other therapies.

3. **BPC-157**: This synthetic peptide has demonstrated anti-inflammatory and tissue-repair properties. BPC-157 modulates the production of pro-inflammatory cytokines, reducing inflammation and promoting healing. It has shown potential in the treatment of inflammatory bowel disease, tendon injuries, and other conditions associated with chronic pain.

4. **Thymosin Beta-4**: Known for its role in tissue repair and regeneration, thymosin beta-4 promotes the migration and differentiation of nerve cells, facilitating nerve regeneration. It has shown promise in the treatment of neuropathic pain and nerve injuries, helping to restore normal function and reduce pain.

5. **Substance P Antagonists**: Substance P is a key neurotransmitter involved in pain transmission and inflammation. Peptides that act as substance P antagonists can block its effects, reducing pain and inflammation.

Research into substance P antagonists has led to the development of potential treatments for conditions like arthritis and fibromyalgia.

6. **KPV (Lys-Pro-Val)**: KPV is a tripeptide derived from the alpha-melanocyte-stimulating hormone (α-MSH). It has been found to possess potent anti-inflammatory properties and can inhibit the release of pro-inflammatory cytokines. KPV shows promise in reducing pain and inflammation in conditions such as inflammatory bowel disease and other inflammatory disorders.

These examples highlight the diverse mechanisms by which peptides can modulate pain pathways, offering targeted and effective solutions for chronic pain management. The specificity of peptide actions reduces the likelihood of side effects and makes them an attractive option for patients who have not found relief with conventional treatments.

Chapter 4

Reducing Inflammation with Peptides

Chronic inflammation is a silent yet pervasive condition that underlies numerous diseases, contributing to the global burden of illness. Despite significant advancements in medical science, effectively managing chronic inflammation remains a challenge with traditional therapies often falling short. Peptide therapies, however, offer new hope, presenting a novel approach to modulating inflammatory pathways with precision. In this chapter, we delve into the problem of chronic inflammation, explore anti-inflammatory peptides and their benefits, and review clinical trials and real-world applications of these promising therapies.

The Problem of Chronic Inflammation

Inflammation is a fundamental biological response to injury, infection, or harmful stimuli. It is characterized by redness, swelling, heat, and pain, serving as the body's mechanism to eliminate pathogens, clear damaged cells, and initiate tissue repair. Acute inflammation is typically beneficial, resolving once the threat is neutralized. However, when inflammation persists and becomes chronic, it can lead to a range of health problems.

Chronic inflammation is defined as a prolonged and dysregulated inflammatory response that lasts for months or years. Unlike acute inflammation, which is self-limiting, chronic inflammation involves continuous tissue damage and repair, leading to a cycle of persistent inflammation and injury. This ongoing inflammatory state is associated with several diseases and conditions, including:

1. **Cardiovascular Diseases**: Chronic inflammation plays a crucial role in the development and progression of atherosclerosis, a condition characterized by the buildup of plaques in the arteries. Inflammatory processes contribute to plaque formation, destabilization, and rupture, leading to heart attacks and strokes.

2. **Autoimmune Disorders**: Conditions like rheumatoid arthritis, lupus, and multiple sclerosis are driven by chronic inflammation, where the immune system mistakenly attacks the body's own tissues. This leads to ongoing tissue damage and significant morbidity.

3. **Metabolic Syndrome and Diabetes**: Chronic inflammation is implicated in insulin resistance, a key feature of metabolic syndrome and type 2 diabetes. Inflammatory mediators interfere with insulin signaling, promoting hyperglycemia and other metabolic disturbances.

4. **Neurodegenerative Diseases**: Inflammatory processes in the brain are linked to neurodegenerative conditions such as Alzheimer's disease and Parkinson's disease. Chronic inflammation contributes to neuronal damage and cognitive decline.

5. **Cancer**: Inflammation is a recognized hallmark of cancer, playing a role in tumor initiation, progression, and metastasis. Chronic inflammatory states create a microenvironment conducive to cancer cell survival and proliferation.

6. **Inflammatory Bowel Disease (IBD):** Chronic inflammation of the gastrointestinal tract, as seen in Crohn's disease and ulcerative colitis, leads to severe symptoms and complications, including increased risk of colorectal cancer.

Challenges in Treating Chronic Inflammation with Traditional Therapies

Traditional therapies for chronic inflammation primarily involve the use of nonsteroidal anti-inflammatory drugs (NSAIDs), corticosteroids, and disease-modifying antirheumatic drugs (DMARDs). While these treatments can be effective, they come with several limitations and challenges:

1. **Side Effects**: Long-term use of NSAIDs can lead to gastrointestinal bleeding, cardiovascular events, and renal impairment. Corticosteroids, though potent anti-inflammatory agents, are associated with a range of

side effects, including osteoporosis, hyperglycemia, and increased susceptibility to infections.

2. **Limited Efficacy**: In many cases, traditional therapies do not fully control chronic inflammation or its underlying causes. Patients may experience incomplete relief, requiring higher doses or combination therapies that increase the risk of adverse effects.

3. **Tolerance and Resistance**: Over time, patients may develop tolerance to certain anti-inflammatory drugs, necessitating higher doses for the same therapeutic effect. Additionally, some conditions, such as autoimmune diseases, may exhibit resistance to standard treatments.

4. **Non-Specific Targeting**: Traditional anti-inflammatory drugs often have broad mechanisms of action, affecting multiple pathways and leading to unintended consequences. This lack of specificity can result in off-target effects and systemic toxicity.

Given these challenges, there is a pressing need for targeted and effective therapies that can modulate inflammation without causing significant side effects. Peptides, with their ability to interact with specific molecular targets, offer a promising alternative.

Anti-Inflammatory Peptides and Their Benefits

Peptides are short chains of amino acids that play crucial roles in various biological processes, including immune regulation and inflammation. Several peptides have been identified for their potent anti-inflammatory properties, making them attractive candidates for therapeutic development. Notable examples include:

1. **Thymosin Beta-4 (Tβ4):** Thymosin Beta-4 is a naturally occurring peptide involved in tissue repair and regeneration. It exhibits anti-inflammatory effects by reducing the production of pro-inflammatory cytokines and chemokines. Tβ4 also promotes the migration and

differentiation of cells involved in wound healing and has shown promise in treating inflammatory conditions.

2. **Melanocortin Peptides**: Melanocortin peptides, such as α-MSH (alpha-melanocyte-stimulating hormone), are derived from the precursor protein pro-opiomelanocortin (POMC). These peptides have anti-inflammatory and immunomodulatory properties, acting on melanocortin receptors to inhibit the production of pro-inflammatory mediators. α-MSH has been investigated for its potential to treat inflammatory skin conditions and autoimmune diseases.

3. **BPC-157**: BPC-157 is a synthetic peptide derived from a protein found in the stomach. It has demonstrated significant anti-inflammatory effects by modulating the production of inflammatory cytokines and enhancing angiogenesis. BPC-157 has been explored for its potential to promote healing in inflammatory bowel disease, tendon injuries, and other inflammatory conditions.

4. **KPV (Lys-Pro-Val)**: KPV is a tripeptide derived from α-MSH that possesses anti-inflammatory properties. It inhibits the release of pro-inflammatory cytokines and

reduces oxidative stress. KPV has shown potential in treating inflammatory conditions such as inflammatory bowel disease and skin disorders.

5. **Anakinra**: Anakinra is a recombinant form of the human interleukin-1 receptor antagonist (IL-1Ra). It binds to the IL-1 receptor, preventing the binding of the pro-inflammatory cytokine IL-1 and thereby reducing inflammation. Anakinra is used in the treatment of rheumatoid arthritis and other inflammatory conditions.

Anti-inflammatory peptides exert their effects through various mechanisms, targeting specific pathways involved in the inflammatory response. Some of the key mechanisms include:

1. **Inhibition of Pro-Inflammatory Cytokines**: Many anti-inflammatory peptides work by inhibiting the production or activity of pro-inflammatory cytokines such as TNF-α, IL-1, and IL-6. By blocking these cytokines,

peptides can reduce inflammation and tissue damage. For example, thymosin beta-4 decreases the levels of TNF-α and IL-6, mitigating the inflammatory response.

2. **Activation of Anti-Inflammatory Pathways**: Peptides can activate pathways that promote the resolution of inflammation. Melanocortin peptides, such as α-MSH, bind to melanocortin receptors on immune cells, triggering anti-inflammatory signaling cascades. This results in the production of anti-inflammatory mediators like IL-10 and the inhibition of pro-inflammatory pathways.

3. **Modulation of Immune Cell Activity**: Anti-inflammatory peptides can modulate the activity of immune cells involved in the inflammatory response. BPC-157, for example, enhances the migration and differentiation of cells involved in tissue repair, such as fibroblasts and endothelial cells. This promotes the healing of inflamed tissues and reduces chronic inflammation.

4. **Reduction of Oxidative Stress**: Oxidative stress is a key driver of chronic inflammation. Peptides like KPV exhibit antioxidant properties, reducing the levels of reactive oxygen species (ROS) and mitigating oxidative damage.

This helps to attenuate the inflammatory response and protect tissues from further injury.

5. **Blocking Inflammatory Receptors**: Some peptides act as antagonists to specific inflammatory receptors, preventing the binding of pro-inflammatory ligands. Anakinra, for instance, blocks the IL-1 receptor, preventing IL-1 from exerting its pro-inflammatory effects. This reduces inflammation and provides relief in conditions such as rheumatoid arthritis.

The specificity of these mechanisms allows anti-inflammatory peptides to target the underlying causes of chronic inflammation more precisely than traditional therapies. This reduces the risk of side effects and enhances the overall efficacy of treatment.

Clinical Trials and Real-World Applications

The potential of anti-inflammatory peptides has been explored in numerous clinical trials, demonstrating their efficacy in various conditions characterized by chronic inflammation. Some notable trials include:

1. **Thymosin Beta-4 in Wound Healing**: Thymosin Beta-4 has been investigated for its role in promoting wound healing and reducing inflammation. Clinical trials have shown that Tβ4 can accelerate the healing of chronic wounds, such as diabetic ulcers and venous leg ulcers, by reducing inflammation and enhancing tissue repair.

2. **Melanocortin Peptides in Autoimmune Diseases**: Clinical studies have explored the use of melanocortin peptides, such as α-MSH, in the treatment of autoimmune diseases. For example, a trial investigating the effects of α-MSH in patients with inflammatory bowel disease demonstrated a significant reduction in disease activity and inflammatory markers, highlighting its potential as a therapeutic agent.

3. **BPC-157 in Inflammatory Bowel Disease**: BPC-157 has shown promise in preclinical and clinical studies for the treatment of inflammatory bowel disease (IBD). Clinical trials have reported improvements in mucosal healing,

reduction in inflammatory cytokines, and overall symptom relief in patients with IBD. These findings suggest that BPC-157 may offer a novel and effective approach to managing chronic inflammation in the gastrointestinal tract.

4. **Anakinra in Rheumatoid Arthritis**: Anakinra has been extensively studied in the context of rheumatoid arthritis. Clinical trials have demonstrated that Anakinra effectively reduces joint inflammation, pain, and swelling in patients with rheumatoid arthritis by blocking IL-1 signaling. Its use has also been explored in other inflammatory conditions, including systemic juvenile idiopathic arthritis and gout.

Practical Application of These Peptides in Clinical Settings and Everyday Use.

The translation of anti-inflammatory peptides from clinical trials to real-world applications involves several considerations, including safety, efficacy, and practical aspects of administration. The following sections highlight how these peptides are being integrated into clinical practice and everyday use:

1. **Safety and Efficacy**: Safety is paramount in the use of any therapeutic agent. Anti-inflammatory peptides have generally shown favorable safety profiles in clinical trials, with fewer side effects compared to traditional anti-inflammatory drugs. However, long-term safety data are still needed for some peptides, and ongoing monitoring is essential. Efficacy is also a critical factor, and real-world evidence from clinical practice will continue to inform the optimal use of these peptides.

2. **Administration and Dosage**: The route of administration and dosage of anti-inflammatory peptides can vary depending on the peptide and the condition being treated. Injectable peptides, such as BPC-157 and thymosin beta-4, are typically administered subcutaneously or intramuscularly. Advances in peptide delivery systems are expanding the options for administration, including transdermal patches and oral formulations, which can enhance patient compliance and convenience.

3. **Combination Therapies**: In many cases, anti-inflammatory peptides can be used in combination

with other treatments to achieve synergistic effects. For example, combining peptides with conventional anti-inflammatory drugs, physical therapy, or lifestyle modifications may enhance overall outcomes. Personalized treatment plans that consider the patient's specific condition, response to therapy, and preferences are crucial for optimizing results.

4. **Monitoring and Follow-Up**: Regular monitoring and follow-up are essential to assess the effectiveness of peptide therapies and adjust treatment as needed. Healthcare providers should track clinical outcomes, inflammatory markers, and any potential side effects. Patient education and engagement are also important, as patients play a key role in managing their condition and adhering to therapy.

5. **Accessibility and Cost**: The cost and accessibility of anti-inflammatory peptides can influence their use in clinical practice. While some peptides are commercially available and covered by insurance, others may be more expensive or require compounding by specialized pharmacies. Efforts to improve accessibility and

affordability, including research into cost-effective production methods, are ongoing.

6. **Patient Selection**: Identifying the right candidates for peptide therapy is critical. Not all patients with chronic inflammation will benefit equally from these treatments. Factors such as the underlying cause of inflammation, disease severity, and previous treatment history should be considered. Genetic and biomarker testing may also help to identify patients who are likely to respond well to peptide therapy.

7. **Regulatory Considerations**: The regulatory landscape for peptide therapies is evolving. Regulatory agencies, such as the FDA and EMA, assess the safety and efficacy of new peptide treatments before approval. Clinicians and patients should stay informed about the regulatory status of specific peptides and any emerging guidelines or recommendations.

Chapter 5

Peptides and Anti-Aging

Aging is a natural and inevitable process that affects every living organism. It is characterized by a gradual decline in physiological functions, increased susceptibility to diseases, and a reduction in the capacity to respond to stress. Understanding the science of aging involves exploring the biological mechanisms that drive these changes and identifying the factors that contribute to the aging process.

At the cellular level, aging is marked by several key phenomena:

1. **Cellular Senescence**: This is the process by which cells cease to divide and function effectively. Senescent cells accumulate in tissues over time, secreting inflammatory

factors that can damage neighboring cells and contribute to tissue dysfunction.

2. **Telomere Shortening****: Telomeres are protective caps at the ends of chromosomes that shorten with each cell division. When telomeres become critically short, cells enter a state of senescence or undergo apoptosis (programmed cell death).

3. **Mitochondrial Dysfunction**: Mitochondria, the powerhouses of the cell, produce energy in the form of ATP. As we age, mitochondrial function declines, leading to reduced energy production and increased oxidative stress, which can damage cellular components.

4. **DNA Damage and Repair**: Accumulation of DNA damage over time, coupled with a decline in the efficiency of DNA repair mechanisms, can lead to mutations and cellular dysfunction.

5. **Epigenetic Changes**: Epigenetic modifications, such as DNA methylation and histone modification, influence gene expression without altering the underlying DNA sequence. Age-related changes in the epigenome can disrupt normal cellular functions.

6. **Loss of Proteostasis**: The maintenance of protein homeostasis (proteostasis) involves the synthesis, folding, and degradation of proteins. Aging impairs proteostasis, leading to the accumulation of damaged and misfolded proteins.

Systemically, aging manifests in various ways:

1. **Skin Aging**: The skin becomes thinner, less elastic, and more prone to wrinkles and age spots due to reduced collagen production and increased degradation of extracellular matrix components.

2. **Musculoskeletal Decline**: There is a loss of muscle mass and strength (sarcopenia), decreased bone density (osteoporosis), and joint stiffness, contributing to frailty and reduced mobility.

3. **Cognitive Decline**: Aging is associated with changes in brain structure and function, leading to cognitive impairments such as memory loss and reduced processing speed.

4. **Immune System Aging (Immunosenescence)**: The immune system becomes less effective with age, resulting in increased susceptibility to infections, reduced response to vaccines, and a higher incidence of autoimmune diseases.

5. **Cardiovascular Aging**: The risk of cardiovascular diseases, such as hypertension, atherosclerosis, and heart failure, increases with age due to changes in blood vessels and heart function.

Peptides That Promote Longevity and Vitality

Research has identified several peptides that show promise in slowing the aging process and promoting longevity and vitality. These peptides work through various mechanisms to enhance cellular function, reduce inflammation, and support tissue repair and regeneration.

1. **Human Growth Hormone (HGH) and Growth Hormone-Releasing Peptides (GHRPs)**:

   - **HGH**: Human growth hormone stimulates growth, cell reproduction, and regeneration. It plays a crucial role in maintaining muscle mass, bone density, and metabolic function. Synthetic HGH and peptides that stimulate its release (e.g., sermorelin, ipamorelin) are used to counteract age-related decline in HGH levels.

   - **GHRPs**: These peptides mimic the effects of ghrelin, a hormone that stimulates the release of growth hormone from the pituitary gland. Examples include GHRP-2, GHRP-6, and hexarelin.

2. **Thymosin Alpha-1 (Tα1):**

   - Thymosin alpha-1 is a peptide derived from the thymus gland. It enhances immune function, reduces inflammation, and has been shown to have anti-aging effects by promoting cellular repair and regeneration.

3. **Epitalon**:

- Epitalon (Epithalon) is a synthetic version of a naturally occurring peptide called epithalamin, produced by the pineal gland. It has been shown to lengthen telomeres, improve sleep, and enhance the function of the endocrine and immune systems, thereby promoting longevity.

4. **BPC-157**:

- BPC-157 is a peptide derived from gastric juice. It has potent healing and regenerative properties, promoting tissue repair, reducing inflammation, and protecting against the harmful effects of oxidative stress.

5. **Thymosin Beta-4 (Tβ4)**:

- Thymosin beta-4 plays a key role in tissue repair and regeneration. It promotes wound healing, reduces inflammation, and supports angiogenesis (formation of new blood vessels).

6. **Collagen Peptides**:

- Collagen is the most abundant protein in the body, providing structural support to the skin, joints, and connective tissues. Supplementing with collagen peptides can improve skin elasticity, reduce wrinkles, and support joint health.

Practical Tips for Using Peptides to Slow Aging

Incorporating anti-aging peptides into daily routines requires careful consideration of factors such as dosage, administration methods, and complementary lifestyle practices. Here are practical guidelines to help maximize the benefits of peptide therapies:

1. **Consult with a Healthcare Professional**:

- Before starting any peptide therapy, consult with a healthcare professional experienced in peptide treatments. They can help determine the most appropriate peptides for your specific needs, monitor your progress, and adjust dosages as necessary.

2. Understand the Administration Methods:

- Peptides can be administered in various forms, including subcutaneous injections, oral supplements, transdermal patches, and topical creams. The choice of administration method depends on the peptide and the desired effects. For example, HGH and GHRPs are commonly administered via subcutaneous injection, while collagen peptides are typically taken orally.

3. Follow Recommended Dosages:

- Adhering to the recommended dosages is crucial for achieving optimal results and minimizing the risk of side effects. Your healthcare provider will provide guidance on the appropriate dosage based on your age, health status, and treatment goals.

4. **Monitor Progress and Adjust as Needed**:

- Regular monitoring of your progress is essential to ensure the effectiveness of the peptide therapy. Keep track of any changes in your physical health, energy levels, and overall well-being. Adjustments to the treatment plan may be necessary based on your response to the peptides.

5. **Combine Peptide Therapy with a Healthy Lifestyle**:

- Peptide therapy is most effective when combined with a healthy lifestyle. Incorporate the following practices to enhance the anti-aging effects of peptides:

- **Balanced Diet**: Consume a nutrient-rich diet that includes plenty of fruits, vegetables, lean proteins, healthy fats, and whole grains. Nutrients such as antioxidants, vitamins, and minerals support cellular health and combat oxidative stress.

- **Regular Exercise**: Engage in regular physical activity to maintain muscle mass, bone density, and cardiovascular health. Incorporate a mix of aerobic exercises, strength training, and flexibility exercises.

- **Adequate Sleep**: Prioritize sleep to allow your body to repair and regenerate. Aim for 7-9 hours of quality sleep per night.

- **Stress Management**: Practice stress-reducing techniques such as mindfulness meditation, yoga, deep breathing exercises, and hobbies that bring joy and relaxation.

- **Hydration**: Stay well-hydrated to support cellular function and overall health. Drink plenty of water throughout the day.

6. **Protect Your Skin**:

- The skin is often the first area to show signs of aging. Protect your skin from environmental damage by using sunscreen with broad-spectrum protection, wearing protective clothing, and avoiding excessive sun exposure. Incorporate skincare products that contain peptides, antioxidants, and hydrating ingredients.

7. **Avoid Harmful Habits**:

- Minimize or eliminate habits that accelerate aging, such as smoking, excessive alcohol consumption, and a sedentary lifestyle. These behaviors can contribute to oxidative stress, inflammation, and cellular damage.

8. **Stay Informed**:

- The field of peptide therapy is continuously evolving, with ongoing research and new developments. Stay informed about the latest advancements in peptide science and anti-aging treatments. Attend conferences, read scientific literature, and engage with healthcare professionals to keep up-to-date with emerging trends.

Chapter 6

Peptide Therapy Protocols

Starting with peptide therapies can be an exciting and transformative journey toward improved health and wellness. However, it requires careful planning, professional guidance, and informed decision-making to ensure safety and efficacy. Here, we offer a step-by-step guide to help you begin your peptide therapy journey.

Step-by-Step Instructions for Beginning Peptide Therapy

1. **Consult with Healthcare Providers**:

- The first and most crucial step is to consult with a healthcare provider experienced in peptide therapies. This could be a physician, endocrinologist, or a specialist in regenerative medicine. A qualified healthcare provider will assess your overall health, discuss your goals, and determine if peptide therapy is suitable for you.

- During the consultation, be prepared to provide a detailed medical history, including any chronic conditions, medications, allergies, and previous treatments. This information is essential for tailoring a peptide therapy plan to your specific needs.

2. **Initial Assessments and Considerations**:

- **Comprehensive Blood Work**: Your healthcare provider will likely order a series of blood tests to assess your hormonal balance, immune function, and other relevant biomarkers. These tests provide baseline data and help identify any underlying issues that may need to be addressed before starting peptide therapy.

- **Diagnostic Imaging**: In some cases, diagnostic imaging such as MRIs or ultrasounds may be necessary to evaluate specific conditions or monitor the effects of peptide therapy on targeted tissues.

- **Lifestyle Assessment**: Your healthcare provider may also evaluate your diet, exercise habits, stress levels, and sleep patterns. Lifestyle factors play a significant role in the effectiveness of peptide therapy and overall health outcomes.

3. Setting Realistic Goals:

- Discuss your health and wellness goals with your healthcare provider. Whether you aim to alleviate chronic pain, reduce inflammation, improve skin health, or enhance athletic performance, setting clear and realistic goals is essential. Your provider will help you understand what to expect from peptide therapy and set achievable milestones.

4. Choosing the Right Peptides:

- Based on your health assessment and goals, your healthcare provider will recommend specific peptides that align with your needs. Different peptides have unique mechanisms of action and benefits, so selecting the right ones is critical for success.

5. **Personalized Treatment Plan**:

- Your healthcare provider will create a personalized treatment plan that includes the types of peptides, dosages, administration methods, and duration of therapy. The plan will also outline any necessary lifestyle adjustments to complement the peptide therapy.

6. **Education and Informed Consent**:

- Before starting peptide therapy, ensure you fully understand the treatment, including potential benefits, risks, and side effects. Your healthcare provider should provide educational materials and answer any questions you may have. Informed consent is an important step to ensure you are comfortable and confident in your decision.

Dosage Guidelines and Administration Methods

Proper dosage and administration of peptides are crucial to maximizing their benefits and minimizing potential side effects. Here, we provide detailed dosage recommendations and explain the various methods of peptide administration.

Dosage Recommendations for Different Peptides and Conditions

1. Human Growth Hormone (HGH) and Growth Hormone-Releasing Peptides (GHRPs):

- **HGH**: The typical starting dose for HGH therapy is 1-2 IU (international units) per day, administered subcutaneously. The dosage may be adjusted based on individual response and goals, with a typical range of 1-4 IU per day. HGH is often used for anti-aging, muscle growth, and fat loss.

- **GHRPs**: Common GHRPs include sermorelin, ipamorelin, and GHRP-2. Dosages vary depending on the peptide, but a general guideline is 100-300 mcg (micrograms) per day, administered subcutaneously. GHRPs stimulate the release of endogenous growth hormone and are often used in combination with HGH for enhanced effects.

2. Thymosin Alpha-1 (Tα1):

- Thymosin Alpha-1 is typically dosed at 1.6 mg (milligrams) twice weekly, administered subcutaneously. It is used to boost immune function, reduce inflammation, and support recovery from infections and autoimmune conditions.

3. Epitalon:

- Epitalon is usually administered in cycles, with a typical dose of 10 mg per day for 10-20 days, followed by a break period. It is administered subcutaneously and is used for anti-aging, improving sleep quality, and enhancing overall vitality.

4. **BPC-157**:

- BPC-157 is dosed at 200-500 mcg per day, administered subcutaneously or intramuscularly. It is used for its healing properties, promoting tissue repair, and reducing inflammation. The dosage may vary based on the severity of the condition being treated.

5. **Thymosin Beta-4 (Tβ4):**

- Thymosin Beta-4 is typically dosed at 2-5 mg per week, administered subcutaneously. It is used to accelerate wound healing, reduce inflammation, and support tissue regeneration.

6. **Collagen Peptides**:

- Collagen peptides are usually taken orally in doses ranging from 10-20 grams per day. They are used to improve skin elasticity, support joint health, and promote overall tissue repair.

Methods of Peptide Administration and Their Advantages and Disadvantages

1. **Subcutaneous Injection**:

- **Description**: Subcutaneous injections involve injecting peptides into the fatty tissue just beneath the skin using a small needle.

- **Advantages**:

  - High bioavailability, ensuring efficient absorption of the peptide.

  - Allows for precise dosage control.

  - Minimizes gastrointestinal degradation, preserving peptide integrity.

- **Disadvantages**:

  - Requires self-administration or administration by a healthcare provider.

- Potential for injection site reactions such as redness or swelling.

2. **Intramuscular Injection**:

- **Description**: Intramuscular injections involve injecting peptides directly into muscle tissue using a slightly larger needle.

- **Advantages**:

  - Rapid absorption into the bloodstream.

  - Suitable for larger volumes of peptides.

  - Can target specific muscles for localized effects.

- **Disadvantages**:

  - Requires skill and precision to avoid injury.

  - Potential for muscle soreness or discomfort at the injection site.

3. **Oral Administration**:

- **Description**: Oral administration involves taking peptides in the form of capsules, tablets, or powders.

- **Advantages**:

  - Convenient and non-invasive.

  - Ideal for peptides that are stable in the digestive tract, such as collagen peptides.

- **Disadvantages**:

  - Lower bioavailability due to degradation by stomach acid and digestive enzymes.

  - Higher doses may be required to achieve therapeutic effects.

4. **Transdermal Delivery**:

- Description: Transdermal delivery involves applying peptides to the skin using patches, creams, or gels.

- **Advantages**:

  - Non-invasive and easy to use.

- Provides sustained release of peptides over time.

   - Bypasses the digestive system, preserving peptide integrity.

- **Disadvantages**:

   - Variable absorption rates depending on skin type and condition.

   - Potential for skin irritation or allergic reactions.

5. **Intranasal Administration**:

- **Description**: Intranasal administration involves spraying peptides into the nasal cavity using a nasal spray or drops.

- **Advantages**:

   - Rapid absorption through the nasal mucosa.

   - Bypasses the digestive system and hepatic metabolism.

   - Convenient and non-invasive.

- **Disadvantages**:

- Limited to small peptide molecules.

- Potential for nasal irritation or discomfort.

6. **Topical Application**:

- **Description**: Topical application involves applying peptides directly to the skin using creams, lotions, or serums.

- **Advantages**:

- Non-invasive and easy to apply.

- Suitable for localized treatment of skin conditions.

- Can be combined with other skincare ingredients.

- **Disadvantages**:

- Limited penetration into deeper skin layers.

- Variable absorption rates depending on skin type and condition.

To ensure the success of peptide therapy, it is essential to follow best practices and guidelines for safe and effective use. Here are some key considerations:

1. **Maintain Sterility**:

- When administering peptides via injection, it is crucial to maintain sterility to prevent infections. Use sterile needles and syringes, and follow proper injection techniques. Clean the injection site with an alcohol swab before administering the peptide.

2. **Rotate Injection Sites**:

- To minimize the risk of injection site reactions and tissue damage, rotate injection sites regularly. Common injection sites include the abdomen, thigh, and upper arm.

3. **Store Peptides Properly**:

- Peptides are sensitive to temperature and light, so proper storage is essential to maintain their potency. Store peptides in the refrigerator at the recommended temperature and protect them from light exposure. Avoid freezing peptides unless specified by the manufacturer.

4. **Monitor for Side Effects**:

- While peptides are generally well-tolerated, some individuals may experience side effects such as injection site reactions, headaches, or gastrointestinal disturbances. Monitor your body's response to peptide therapy and report any adverse effects to your healthcare provider.

5. **Adhere to Treatment Plan**:

- Consistency is key to achieving the desired outcomes with peptide therapy. Adhere to the prescribed treatment plan, including dosage, administration frequency, and duration of therapy. Skipping doses or discontinuing therapy prematurely may reduce the effectiveness of the treatment.

6. **Combine with Healthy Lifestyle Practices**:

- Peptide therapy is most effective when combined with a healthy lifestyle. Maintain a balanced diet, engage in regular physical activity, manage stress, and prioritize sleep. These practices enhance the overall benefits of peptide therapy and support long-term health and wellness.

7. **Regular Follow-Up Appointments**:

- Schedule regular follow-up appointments with your healthcare provider to monitor your progress and make any necessary adjustments to your peptide therapy plan. Regular assessments ensure that the treatment remains effective and allows for early detection of any potential issues.

8. **Educate Yourself**:

- Stay informed about peptide therapies by reading scientific literature, attending workshops or seminars, and participating in online forums or support groups. Being knowledgeable about the therapies you are using empowers you to make informed decisions and actively participate in your health management.

Chapter 7

Safety and Efficacy of Peptide Treatments

Peptide therapies are increasingly popular for their potential health benefits, but as with any medical treatment, safety and efficacy are paramount. This chapter explores the potential side effects of peptide therapies, strategies for mitigating these side effects, understanding contraindications and precautions, and ensuring the quality and purity of peptide products.

Potential Side Effects and How to Mitigate Them

While peptide therapies are generally well-tolerated, they can sometimes cause side effects. Understanding these side effects and knowing how to manage them can help you have a positive experience with peptide therapy.

Common Side Effects Associated with Peptide Therapies:

1. **Injection Site Reactions**:

 - **Description**: Redness, swelling, pain, or irritation at the injection site are common.

 - **Mitigation**: Use proper injection techniques, rotate injection sites, and use sterile equipment. Applying ice or a cold pack to the site before and after injection can reduce swelling and pain.

2. **Headaches**:

 - **Description**: Some individuals may experience headaches when starting peptide therapy.

 - **Mitigation**: Stay hydrated and ensure you are getting enough sleep. If headaches persist, consult your healthcare provider to adjust the dosage or frequency of injections.

3. Nausea and Gastrointestinal Issues:

- **Description**: Nausea, bloating, or gastrointestinal discomfort may occur.

- **Mitigation**: Taking peptides with food can help minimize gastrointestinal issues. If symptoms persist, speak with your healthcare provider about adjusting your dosage.

4. Fatigue:

- **Description**: Some people may feel unusually tired or fatigued after starting peptide therapy.

- **Mitigation**: Ensure you are getting adequate rest and nutrition. If fatigue persists, discuss with your healthcare provider to adjust your treatment plan.

5. Hormonal Imbalances:

- **Description**: Peptides that influence hormone levels can sometimes cause hormonal imbalances.

- **Mitigation**: Regular monitoring of hormone levels through blood tests can help detect and address imbalances early. Your healthcare provider can adjust your treatment plan as needed.

6. Allergic Reactions:

- **Description**: Although rare, some individuals may have allergic reactions to peptides.

- **Mitigation**: Conduct a patch test before starting full therapy and report any signs of allergic reactions, such as hives, itching, or difficulty breathing, to your healthcare provider immediately.

Understanding Contraindications and Precautions

Peptide therapies, while beneficial for many, may not be suitable for everyone. Understanding contraindications and taking necessary precautions can prevent adverse effects and ensure safe use.

Conditions and Situations Where Peptide Therapies May Not Be Appropriate:

1. **Autoimmune Diseases**:

   - **Description**: Some peptides can stimulate the immune system, which may exacerbate autoimmune conditions.

   - **Precaution**: Patients with autoimmune diseases should consult their healthcare provider before starting peptide therapy.

2. **Cancer**:

   - **Description**: Certain peptides may influence cell growth and proliferation, which could be problematic for cancer patients.

   - **Precaution**: Peptide therapy is generally contraindicated in active cancer cases. Cancer patients or survivors should seek advice from an oncologist before considering peptide treatments.

3. **Pregnancy and Breastfeeding**:

   - **Description**: The safety of peptide therapies during pregnancy and breastfeeding is not well-studied.

   - **Precaution**: Pregnant or breastfeeding women should avoid peptide therapies unless approved by their healthcare provider.

4. **Severe Kidney or Liver Disease**:

   - **Description**: These conditions can affect the body's ability to metabolize and excrete peptides.

   - **Precaution**: Patients with severe kidney or liver disease should be closely monitored by their healthcare provider when undergoing peptide therapy.

Guidelines for Safe Use of Peptides in Different Populations:

1. **Elderly Patients**:

   - **Considerations**: Elderly patients may have slower metabolism and different hormone levels.

   - **Guidelines**: Start with lower doses and adjust gradually under medical supervision. Monitor for side effects closely.

2. **Athletes**:

   - **Considerations**: Athletes may use peptides for performance enhancement.

   - **Guidelines**: Ensure peptides are permitted under sports regulations and do not pose health risks. Regular health check-ups are essential.

3. **Children and Adolescents**:

- Considerations: The safety of peptide therapy in young individuals is not well-established.

- Guidelines: Peptide therapy should only be considered under strict medical supervision for specific conditions and with thorough risk-benefit analysis.

Ensuring Quality and Purity of Peptide Products

The quality and purity of peptide products are crucial for their safety and efficacy. Using substandard or contaminated peptides can lead to adverse effects and reduce the effectiveness of the therapy.

The Importance of Sourcing High-Quality Peptides:

1. Ensuring Efficacy:

- High-quality peptides are manufactured under stringent conditions, ensuring their potency and effectiveness. Using low-quality peptides can result in suboptimal therapeutic outcomes.

2. **Safety Concerns**:

- Contaminated or impure peptides can cause serious health issues. Ensuring that peptides are free from contaminants and manufactured in clean environments is vital for patient safety.

Tips for Verifying the Authenticity and Purity of Peptide Products:

1. **Choose Reputable Suppliers**:

- Purchase peptides from well-known and reputable suppliers with a track record of providing high-quality products. Avoid unknown or dubious sources.

2. Check for Third-Party Testing:

- Reputable suppliers often provide certificates of analysis (COAs) from third-party laboratories. These COAs verify the purity, potency, and quality of the peptides.

3. Verify GMP Certification:

- Ensure that the supplier adheres to Good Manufacturing Practices (GMP). GMP certification indicates that the peptides are manufactured in a controlled and standardized environment.

4. Research and Reviews:

- Conduct thorough research on the supplier and read customer reviews. Positive reviews and testimonials from other users can provide insights into the quality of the products.

5. **Packaging and Labeling**:

- High-quality peptides are usually packaged in sterile, tamper-evident vials or containers. Ensure the packaging is intact and labels contain essential information, including batch numbers and expiration dates.

6. **Consult Your Healthcare Provider**:

- Before purchasing peptides, consult your healthcare provider for recommendations on trusted suppliers. They may have preferred suppliers or be able to source peptides on your behalf.

Chapter 8

Future Directions in Peptide Research

Peptide research has come a long way, opening new frontiers in medical science and therapeutic applications. This chapter delves into the exciting future of peptide research, focusing on emerging peptides and their potential uses, and advances in peptide engineering and biotechnology.

Emerging Peptides and Their Potential Uses

As peptide research continues to advance, new and experimental peptides are being discovered and explored for their potential therapeutic benefits. These emerging peptides hold promise for a range of health applications, from treating chronic diseases to enhancing overall wellness.

New and Experimental Peptides:

1. BPC-157:

 - **Overview**: BPC-157 (Body Protection Compound-157) is a synthetic peptide derived from a protective protein found in the stomach. It is being researched for its regenerative and healing properties.

 - **Potential Uses**: Studies suggest that BPC-157 may aid in the healing of tendons, ligaments, and muscles, as well as promoting gut health and reducing inflammation. Its ability to accelerate wound healing and repair damaged tissues makes it a promising candidate for treating injuries and chronic conditions.

2. Thymosin Alpha-1:

 - **Overview**: Thymosin Alpha-1 is a naturally occurring peptide involved in the immune response. It is being studied for its potential to modulate the immune system and enhance immune function.

- **Potential Uses**: This peptide shows promise in boosting the immune system, making it potentially useful in treating infections, autoimmune diseases, and certain types of cancer. Thymosin Alpha-1's ability to enhance the body's natural defense mechanisms positions it as a valuable tool in immunotherapy.

3. **Selank**:

- **Overview**: Selank is a synthetic peptide derived from the naturally occurring peptide tuftsin. It is being researched for its anxiolytic (anxiety-reducing) and cognitive-enhancing effects.

- **Potential Uses**: Selank has shown potential in reducing anxiety, improving mood, and enhancing cognitive functions such as memory and learning. Its ability to regulate neurotransmitter levels in the brain makes it a promising candidate for treating anxiety disorders, depression, and cognitive decline.

4. Epithalon:

- **Overview**: Epithalon is a synthetic version of the naturally occurring peptide epithalamin, produced by the pineal gland. It is being studied for its anti-aging and longevity-promoting effects.

- **Potential Uses**: Research suggests that Epithalon may enhance telomerase activity, leading to longer telomeres and improved cellular health. This peptide's potential to delay the aging process and promote longevity has garnered significant interest in the field of anti-aging medicine.

5. DSIP (Delta Sleep-Inducing Peptide):

- **Overview**: DSIP is a naturally occurring peptide that influences sleep and stress response. It is being explored for its potential to regulate sleep patterns and reduce stress.

- **Potential Uses**: DSIP has shown promise in improving sleep quality, managing stress, and alleviating symptoms of insomnia. Its ability to modulate the body's natural sleep-wake cycle makes it a potential therapeutic option for individuals with sleep disorders and stress-related conditions.

Advances in Peptide Engineering and Biotechnology

The field of peptide engineering and biotechnology is rapidly evolving, leading to significant advancements in peptide synthesis, delivery, and therapeutic applications. These innovations are expanding the possibilities for peptide therapies, making them more effective, targeted, and accessible.

1. **Peptide Stapling**:

   - **Overview**: Peptide stapling is a technique used to enhance the stability and bioavailability of peptides. By introducing chemical cross-links, or "staples," into the peptide structure, researchers can improve its resistance to degradation and increase its half-life in the body.

- **Benefits**: Stapled peptides exhibit improved binding affinity to their target receptors, enhanced stability in biological environments, and prolonged therapeutic effects. This technique is particularly useful for developing peptides with applications in cancer therapy and other chronic diseases.

2. Peptide-Drug Conjugates (PDCs):

- **Overview**: Peptide-drug conjugates (PDCs) are a novel approach to targeted drug delivery. By conjugating therapeutic peptides with small molecule drugs, researchers can achieve precise delivery of drugs to specific cells or tissues.

- **Benefits**: PDCs offer the advantages of targeted therapy, minimizing off-target effects and reducing systemic toxicity. This approach is being explored for treating cancer, infectious diseases, and other conditions where targeted drug delivery can enhance therapeutic outcomes.

3. **Peptide-Based Vaccines**:

- **Overview**: Peptide-based vaccines use short peptide sequences to elicit an immune response against specific pathogens or diseases. This approach is being investigated for its potential to develop vaccines that are safe, effective, and easy to produce.

- **Benefits**: Peptide-based vaccines offer advantages such as ease of synthesis, stability, and the ability to target specific epitopes. They are being explored for preventing infectious diseases, cancer, and autoimmune disorders.

4. **Peptide Nanoparticles**:

- **Overview**: Peptide nanoparticles are engineered particles that encapsulate peptides for improved delivery and controlled release. These nanoparticles can enhance the bioavailability and stability of peptides in the body.

- **Benefits**: Peptide nanoparticles offer targeted delivery to specific cells or tissues, prolonged release profiles, and protection from enzymatic degradation. This technology is being explored for applications in cancer therapy, regenerative medicine, and chronic disease management.

Expanding the Possibilities for Peptide Therapies:

1. Personalized Peptide Therapies:

   - **Overview**: Advances in genomics and proteomics are paving the way for personalized peptide therapies tailored to an individual's genetic makeup and specific health needs.

   - **Benefits:** Personalized peptide therapies offer the potential for highly targeted and effective treatments, reducing the risk of adverse reactions and optimizing therapeutic outcomes. This approach is being explored for conditions such as cancer, autoimmune diseases, and metabolic disorders.

2. Peptide Libraries and High-Throughput Screening:

- **Overview**: The development of extensive peptide libraries and high-throughput screening techniques allows researchers to rapidly identify peptides with specific therapeutic properties.

- **Benefits**: These technologies enable the discovery of novel peptides with potential applications in a wide range of diseases and conditions. High-throughput screening accelerates the process of peptide discovery and optimization, leading to more efficient development of new therapies.

3. **CRISPR and Gene Editing**:

- **Overview**: The integration of peptide engineering with gene editing technologies like CRISPR is opening new avenues for therapeutic interventions. Peptides can be designed to modulate gene expression and repair genetic mutations.

- **Benefits**: Combining peptides with gene editing tools offers the potential for precise and targeted gene therapies, addressing the root causes of genetic diseases. This approach is being explored for treating genetic disorders, cancer, and other conditions with a genetic component.

4. **Peptide-Based Biosensors**:

- **Overview**: Peptide-based biosensors are being developed to detect and monitor various biomarkers in real-time. These biosensors utilize peptides to bind specifically to target molecules, enabling accurate detection and measurement.

- **Benefits**: Peptide-based biosensors offer the potential for early diagnosis, real-time monitoring, and personalized health management. They are being explored for applications in diagnostics, disease monitoring, and environmental sensing.

Chapter 9

Practical Guide to Peptide Therapy

Peptide therapy has become a powerful tool in health and wellness, offering targeted solutions for a wide range of conditions. This chapter provides a comprehensive guide to selecting the right peptides for your needs, sourcing them safely, and integrating peptide therapy into your daily health routine.

Finding the Right Peptide for Your Needs

Choosing the appropriate peptide for your specific health goals is a crucial first step in peptide therapy. With a variety of peptides available, each with unique properties and benefits, understanding how to select the right one can optimize your treatment outcomes.

1. **Identify Your Health Goals**:

- **Pain Relief**: For chronic pain management, peptides like BPC-157 and Thymosin Beta-4 are known for their regenerative properties and ability to reduce inflammation.

- **Anti-Aging**: If your goal is to combat signs of aging, peptides such as Epithalon and GHK-Cu can promote cellular rejuvenation and improve skin health.

- **Immune Support**: Thymosin Alpha-1 is a powerful peptide for enhancing immune function and modulating immune responses, making it ideal for those looking to boost their immunity.

- **Muscle Growth and Recovery**: Athletes and fitness enthusiasts may benefit from peptides like Ipamorelin and CJC-1295, which promote muscle growth and accelerate recovery.

2. **Understand the Mechanism of Action**:

- **Peptide Functions**: Different peptides work through various mechanisms, such as stimulating growth hormone release, reducing inflammation, or modulating immune responses. Understanding how a peptide functions can help you choose one that aligns with your health goals.

3. Consider the Evidence:

- **Research and Clinical Studies**: Review scientific literature and clinical studies to understand the efficacy and safety of the peptide you are considering. Look for peptides that have been extensively researched and shown to be effective in treating your specific condition.

4. Consult with Healthcare Professionals:

- **Expert Guidance**: Work with a healthcare provider who specializes in peptide therapy. They can help you assess your health needs, recommend appropriate peptides, and develop a personalized treatment plan.

Factors to Consider When Choosing Peptides:

1. **Safety and Efficacy**:

- Ensure the peptide has a proven safety profile and has demonstrated efficacy in clinical trials or studies.

- Be aware of potential side effects and interactions with other medications or conditions.

2. **Dosage and Administration**:

- Understand the recommended dosage for your specific condition and how the peptide should be administered (e.g., injectable, oral, transdermal).

3. **Duration of Treatment**:

- Determine the optimal duration for peptide therapy. Some peptides may be used short-term for acute conditions, while others may require long-term use for chronic issues.

4. Cost and Accessibility:

- Consider the cost of peptide therapy and whether it is accessible to you. Some peptides may be more expensive or harder to obtain than others.

Where to Source Peptide Treatments

Sourcing high-quality peptides from reputable suppliers is essential for ensuring the safety and effectiveness of your peptide therapy.

1. Pharmacies and Compounding Pharmacies:

- **Licensed Providers**: Pharmacies, particularly compounding pharmacies, can prepare custom peptide formulations prescribed by your healthcare provider. Ensure the pharmacy is licensed and follows strict quality control standards.

2. **Online Peptide Suppliers**:

 - **Research and Reviews**: When purchasing peptides online, choose suppliers with positive reviews and a good reputation. Look for companies that provide detailed product information and transparency about their manufacturing processes.

 - **Third-Party Testing**: Reputable suppliers should offer third-party testing results to verify the purity and potency of their peptides. Avoid suppliers that do not provide this information.

3. **Healthcare Providers and Clinics**:

 - **Professional Guidance**: Some healthcare providers and specialized clinics offer peptide therapies as part of their treatment programs. These providers can ensure you receive high-quality peptides and appropriate medical supervision.

Importance of Working with Healthcare Professionals:

1. Customized Treatment Plans:

   - Healthcare professionals can create personalized peptide therapy plans tailored to your specific health needs and goals.

2. Monitoring and Adjustments:

   - Regular monitoring by a healthcare provider ensures your peptide therapy is effective and safe. They can adjust dosages and administration methods as needed.

3. Addressing Side Effects and Interactions:

   - Healthcare providers can help manage any side effects or interactions with other medications you may be taking, ensuring a safe and effective treatment experience.

Successfully incorporating peptide therapy into your daily life requires careful planning and a commitment to maintaining a healthy lifestyle.

1. **Create a Routine**:

- **Consistency**: Administer your peptide treatments at the same time each day to establish a routine. Consistency is key to maximizing the benefits of peptide therapy.

- **Reminders**: Use alarms or reminders to help you remember your treatment schedule, especially if you are using multiple peptides with different administration times.

2. **Maintain a Healthy Diet**:

- **Nutrient-Rich Foods**: A balanced diet rich in vitamins, minerals, and antioxidants can enhance the effects of peptide therapy. Focus on whole foods, lean proteins, healthy fats, and plenty of fruits and vegetables.

   - **Hydration**: Staying well-hydrated supports overall health and can improve the absorption and efficacy of peptides.

3. Exercise Regularly:

   - **Physical Activity**: Regular exercise can complement the benefits of peptide therapy, especially for peptides aimed at muscle growth, recovery, and anti-aging. Incorporate a mix of aerobic, strength, and flexibility exercises into your routine.

4. Adequate Sleep:

   - **Rest and Recovery**: Quality sleep is crucial for the body's healing and regenerative processes. Aim for 7-9 hours of sleep per night to support the effects of peptide therapy.

5. Stress Management:

- **Relaxation Techniques**: Practices such as meditation, yoga, and deep breathing can help manage stress, which can otherwise negatively impact your health and the effectiveness of peptide treatments.

Complementary Practices and Lifestyle Changes:

1. Supplements and Nutrition:

- **Supportive Supplements**: Consider supplements that support peptide therapy, such as amino acids, vitamins, and minerals. Consult with your healthcare provider to ensure they are appropriate for your needs.

- **Balanced Nutrition**: Focus on a nutrient-dense diet that supports overall health and enhances the efficacy of peptide treatments.

2. **Mind-Body Practices**:

- **Holistic Approaches**: Integrate mind-body practices like mindfulness, meditation, and acupuncture to support overall well-being and complement peptide therapy.

- **Stress Reduction**: Managing stress through these practices can enhance the effectiveness of peptide treatments and improve your overall health.

3. **Regular Health Monitoring**:

- **Track Progress**: Keep a journal or use health tracking apps to monitor your progress with peptide therapy. Record any changes in symptoms, side effects, and overall health.

- **Routine Check-Ups**: Schedule regular check-ups with your healthcare provider to assess the effectiveness of your peptide therapy and make any necessary adjustments.

4. **Stay Informed**:

- **Education**: Stay informed about the latest research and developments in peptide therapy. Attend seminars, read scientific literature, and engage with healthcare communities to keep up-to-date with new findings and advancements.

Incorporating peptide therapy into your health routine can offer significant benefits, but it requires careful planning, professional guidance, and a commitment to maintaining a healthy lifestyle. By selecting the right peptides, sourcing them from reputable suppliers, and integrating them seamlessly into your daily life, you can optimize the therapeutic potential of peptides and enhance your overall health and well-being.

Conclusion

As we reach the conclusion of this comprehensive guide on peptide therapies, it's evident that we stand on the precipice of a transformative era in health and wellness. Peptides, with their targeted mechanisms and diverse applications, offer promising solutions for many of the challenges faced in modern medicine. From managing chronic pain and inflammation to combating the signs of aging, peptides are redefining our approach to health care and personal well-being.

Peptides represent a paradigm shift in therapeutic strategies. Unlike traditional medications that often come with a host of side effects and systemic impacts, peptides offer precision. Their ability to interact specifically with cellular receptors and influence biochemical pathways means they can address root causes rather than just symptoms.

Looking ahead, the future of peptide research is bright. Emerging peptides and advancements in biotechnology promise to unlock new therapeutic possibilities. Innovations in peptide synthesis, delivery systems, and personalized medicine will continue to drive this field forward, offering tailored solutions for individual health needs.

While peptide therapies offer powerful benefits, they are most effective when integrated into a holistic health approach. Maintaining a healthy diet, regular exercise, adequate sleep, and stress management are essential components of overall well-being. Complementary practices such as mindfulness, meditation, and supportive supplements can further enhance the effects of peptide treatments.

As we embrace this new era of health and wellness with peptide therapies, it's important to recognize the potential they hold for transforming lives. Whether addressing chronic conditions, enhancing athletic performance, or promoting longevity, peptides offer a versatile and powerful tool in the quest for optimal health.

The journey through this book has provided a comprehensive understanding of peptide therapies, from their scientific foundations to their practical applications. As you move forward, consider how peptides can play a role in your own health journey. With informed choices, professional guidance, and a commitment to holistic well-being, you can harness the power of peptides to achieve lasting health and vitality.